OCN Exam Practice Test Set B

160 OCN Practice Questions for ONCC OCN Certification

OCN Exam Expert
© 2021-2022
Printed in USA.

Disclaimer

All rights reserved. It is illegal to distribute, reproduce or transmit any part of this book by any means or forms.

ONCC ®, OCN ® are registered trademarks of Oncology Nursing Certification Corporation. They hold no affiliation with this product.

Every effort has been made by the author and editor to ensure correct information in this book. This book is prepared with extreme care to give the best to its readers. However, the author and editor hereby disclaim any liability to any part for any loss, damage caused by errors or omission. Recording, photocopying or any other mechanical or electronic transmission of the book without prior permission of the publisher is not permitted, except in case of critical reviews and certain other non-commercial uses permitted by copyright law.

© Copyright 2021 by OCN Exam Expert. All rights reserved.

Printed in USA.

Summary

OCN Exam Practice Questions.....................7

Answers & Explanation............................50

Why this OCN Questions Book:

We have taken at most care in preparing the practice questions in this book. The following are the highlights of this book which will make you understand why this book is a great guide to study for and clear the OCN Exam.

- Latest & Frequently Asked Questions: Questions are prepared based on the latest curriculum as specified by the ONCC®. The frequently asked questions are given to make you familiarize with the important concepts.

- Clear Explanation for the correct answer: Our explanation to the practice question will help you to improve your reasoning ability and hence you will be able to answer any type of question with ease.

- No last minute surprise: These practice questions and options are designed in a way that matches the OCN ® Exam so that you don't have a feeling of embarrassment when you take the actual exam.

- More weightage, more exploration: Certain concepts like Symptom Management and Palliative Care, Treatment Modalities are given more weightage in the OCN Exam. Hence we have covered more around these topics which will help you to dive deep in the core concepts and easily pass the exam.

- All the question in this book are prepared and reviewed by **Oncology Experts** considering the latest curriculum.

- There is **one set of practice questions** having **160**

questions with answers and explanation for the correct answer

- The questions in this book are prepared on the basis of the following curriculum as specified by ONCC®.

    I. Care Continuum - 19%

    II. Oncology Nursing Practice - 17 %

    III. Treatment Modalities - 19%

    IV. Symptom Management and Palliative Care - 23%

    V. Oncologic Emergencies - 12%

    VI. Psychosocial Dimensions of Care - 10%

- More Weightage, More Number of Questions for that concept. The questions are randomly ordered just as in the actual OCN exam to improve thinking ability.

ALL THE BEST!! YOU WILL SURELY BE AN ONCOLOGY CERTIFIED NURSE

OCN Exam Practice Questions

OCN Exam Practice Questions Set 2

Question 1: What will be the advice of the nurse, when a 64 year old African American patient asks about the prostate screening for her grown sons?
a) A prostate specific antigen test at the age of 45
b) Sulphonyl acid phosphatase at the age of 45
c) A MRI scan at the age of 45
d) An ultrasound guided biopsy of the prostate ate the beginning of age 45

Question 2: The protective equipment that is recommended during the clean-up of the hazardous medical spill is
a) Vinyl surgical gloves
b) Cloth gown
c) Latex gloves
d) Face shield

Question 3: Mathew, a 78 year old patient has been diagnosed with prostate cancer and cardiovascular disease. He has been administered with naproxen twice a day along with a daily dose of acetylsalicylic acid. What will be the instruction given to the patient?
a) To consume every medicine with proper time interval
b) Consulting the physician regarding the addition of cytoprotectants
c) About the increase in swelling during evening times
d) Consumption of medicine only in the empty stomach

Question 4: Among the following, which is termed as the shortest phase of the cell cycle?
a) Mitosis
b) Gap 1
c) Meiosis
d) Prophase

Question 5: Among the following, the early symptoms for increased intracranial pressure is related to?
a) Nausea
b) Decortication
c) Confusion
d) Fatigue

Question 6: Anticipatory Grief, according to the nurse understanding is?
a) Resolved
b) Unacknowledged
c) Unconscious process
d) Short term

Question 7: Despite the use of antiemetics, Megan reports of nausea and vomiting before every chemotherapy. She starts crying and requests to stop the treatment. How will the nurse calms down Megan?
a) By recommending healthcare provider to reduce dosage
b) By suggesting the healthcare provider to stop treatment
c) By explaining that everyone experience nausea and Vomiting
d) By discussing integrative therapy options

Question 8: Which among the following is said to be the suitable integrative modality for the patient who has pain with a platelet count of $12000/mm^3$?
a) Acupuncture
b) Chemotherapy
c) Massage
d) Reiki therapy

Question 9: Rochelle, a 34 year old patient has been diagnosed with breast cancer. Counseling has been given to Rochelle and her partner William regarding contraception before chemotherapy. Which of the following statement ensures adequate understanding by the couple?

a) "I will call my gynecologist to discuss about having my tubes tied."
b) "I will agree to use birth control pills or a reliable barrier method as recommended by my physician."
c) " I don't have to worry about birth control before receiving chemotherapy"
d) "Hormone pills are the easiest and the safest method of birth control."

Question 10: Who is at the greater risk among the following for bone marrow depression after radiation treatment?
a) A 25-year-old patient receiving chemotherapy and radiation for Hodgkin lymphoma
b) A 67-year-old patient who is being treated for basal cell carcinoma of face
c) A 46-year-old patient receiving boost for Lumpectomy site
d) A 58-year-old patient who is receiving radiation for solitary liver metastasis

Question 11: William is taking opioids for pain management. He reported of increased constipation and has started bowel retaining. What is said to be the best time to assist him to sit on a toilet or commode to initiate bowel evacuation?
a) About half an hour after meal
b) Whenever the patient urges to defecate
c) Early in the morning
d) Exactly before going to sleep

Question 12: Michelle, who received cyclophosphamide five years ago for her breast cancer reported about the beginning of bruising and fatigue recently. These symptoms appears to be the suspect for which of the following options?
a) Cardiomyopathy
b) Leukoencephalopathy

c) Secondary leukemia
d) Liver failure

Question 13: What is the major benefit of survivorship care plan?
a) It will be easier to monitor patient regarding side effects
b) It provides a clear idea about the care and surveillance after treatment
c) It allows the patient to make discussion with their oncologist after the completion of treatment.
d) It allows the patient to have medication during chemotherapy

Question 14: After two weeks of chemotherapy, a patient reports bleeding gums and increased bruises even though the patient has normal platelet count. What is appropriate intervention to be done by the nurse?
a) Review the patient's history for prior treatment with ionizing radiation
b) Review the patient's medical report
c) Suggest the patient to have iron rich food
d) Reassure the patient that this symptoms will reduce after few days

Question 15: A patient with prostate cancer experiences metastasis. Which among the following is said to metastasize frequently?
a) Lung
b) Bone
c) Brain
d) Liver

Question 16: Which among the following is considered as a true positive indication from cancer screening?

a) The patient has cancer despite of the negative result
b) The patient doesn't have cancer despite of positive result
c) The individual has cancer
d) The individual has a symptom for future diagnosis of cancer

Question 17: When developing an education program which of the following action must be performed first?
a) Educational methods had to be selected
b) Assess learning needs
c) Determine educational objective
d) Formulating criteria for evaluation

Question 18: A patient refuses to take opioids stating that even pain is a part of life. What will be the nurse response to this statement?
a) Referring pain to chaplain
b) Requesting an evaluation from the pain service
c) Exploring the meaning of pain with the patient
d) Schedule a visit with CanSurmount volunteer

Question 19: Which of the following exemplifies complicated grief as demonstrated by the spouse of the patient who died recently?
a) Avoiding discussion with hospice service
b) Removing all the pictures from the house and refusing to discuss about the descendant
c) Seeking out new organization to join
d) Attending the support group for the family of cancer patients

Question 20: Which of the following medication is given for radiation induced diarrhea?
a) Cetirizine

b) Erythromycin
c) Glutamine
d) Loperamide

Question 21: How does the alkylating agent exert their pressure?
a) By causing the release of toxic free radicals inside the cell and triggering their apoptosis.
b) By binding to the DNA strand which prevents DNA replication and cell division
c) By disrupting folate dependent metabolic process essential for cell replication
d) By attaching to CD52 on the surface of B and T cells that generally result in antibody dependent lysis.

Question 22: What will be the response of the nurse when enquired about the risk of Lymphedema after undergoing breast conservation surgery with sentinel lymph node biopsy procedure and radiation?
a) If there is no development in the first year, then there is no development in the progressive years.
b) Although the risk is low precaution has to be taken
c) There is no occurrence of Lymphedema after sentinel lymph node procedure
d) If Lymphedema guidelines are followed then there will be no occurrence

Question 23: William, a patient with prostate cancer administers oxycodone orally for the relief from pain every 4 hours. A Nurse, while paying a home visit finds that there has been no bowel movement with constant and dull back pain for the past 3 days. These symptoms are likely to indicate?
a) Impending spinal cord compression

b) Adverse effect of oxycodone
c) Excess abdominal fluid (Ascites)
d) Hypocalcemia

Question 24: According to the Buddhist tradition, they believe that a deceased person's body should not be disturbed for at least four hours. The most likely reason behind this might be:
a) The patient's family might need some time to cope-up with the patient's loss.
b) The patient's family may need some time to do the final rituals of the patient for his well-being in the afterlife.
c) They believe that a soul needs some time to leave off the body and be at peace.
d) The person might have been diagnosed with an infectious disease and they might need some time to dispose the body properly.

Question 25: Which of the following has to be administered as initial treatment for the patient with septic shock?
a) Vasopressors
b) IV antibiotics
c) IV antifungals
d) Corticosteroids at high dosage

Question 26: Robert has pulmonary metastasis and has been receiving repeated thoracentesis. Which among the following development will the nurse be more concerned about?
a) Constriction of airways in the lung
b) lung expansion minimization (trapped lung)
c) Lung embolism
d) Pneumonitis

Question 27: Jonas, 62 years old patient with CD33 positive acute myeloid leukemia has a left ejection fraction of 40% during first relapse. What is the treatment suggested for Jonas?
a) Intravenous drug Rituximab
b) Cytosine arbinoside
c) All trans retinoic acids
d) Gemtuzumab ozogamicin

Question 28: What has to be done when Robin reports of yellow, crusted papules and itching of shoulder after a targeted therapy?
a) Using a moisturizer containing retinoid twice a day
b) Apply aloe Vera on the affected region
c) Apply lotion with Dimethicone
d) Dilute hot bath water with half strength Dakin's solution

Question 29: The most prominent symptom of oral mucositis is?
a) Pain
b) Headache
c) Eye Infection
d) Bleeding

Question 30: Which of the following is considered as a modal quality of cancer treatment regarding surgery?
a) It is considered as the only treatment that the patient requires
b) It is used as a palliative measure to relieve symptoms
c) It aims to remove only a portion of tumor
d) It causes less toxicity when used along with chemotherapy

Question 31: Why are certain tumor cells described as undifferentiated cells?
a) Because they resemble normal cells
b) Because they remain in same position
c) Because they grow at a faster rate
d) Because they don't grow

Question 32: David is 70 year old having prostate cancer and vertebral tenderness . He bears so much pain during his bowel movements. He also suffering with muscle loss and sensory paresthesia. The appropriate cause for this is:
a) spinal cord compression
b) loss of urine or bowel control
c) urinary infection
d) Lower Back strain

Question 33: The cells from which oligodendroglia tumors originate maintains the function of ?
a) Cell body
b) Myelin sheath
c) Synovial fluid
d) Pericardial fluid

Question 34: The type of cancer that can develop due to excessive use of smokeless tobacco and alcohol is?
a) Laryngeal cancer
b) Gastric cancer
c) Lymphatic cancer
d) Lung cancer

Question 35: A patient is scheduled to receive oxaliplatin. Which of the following denotes that the patient needs additional teaching?
a) I'm going to eat ice chips while receiving chemotherapy in order to avoid mouth sores.
b) I'll call the triage number if I develop fever
c) I have ordered a wig to match my hair color
d) Before starting my chemotherapy I'm scheduled to get my first flu shot.

Question 36: What is the most common cause of lung cancer?

a) Genetic mutation.
b) Exposure to chemical waste.
c) Exposure to direct or secondary tobacco smoke.
d) Exposure to ultraviolet rays from the sun.

Question 37: Among the following condition of the cancer patient, who is most likely to experience sexual dysfunction?
a) A patient who has a history of marital discord
b) A female patient with hypertension
c) A young and newly married patient
d) A patient and partner who schedule time for their sexual activity.

Question 38: William suddenly got provoked with a doubt while Docetaxel was infused. He asked the nurse why dexamethasone is prescribed. The nurse responds by saying that it prevents ?
a) Fluid retention
b) Anorexia nervosa
c) Sudden uncontrolled electric disturbances
d) Fatigue

Question 39: Among the following, which option can clearly explain the cancer survivorship plan?
a) Outlining about the primary therapies received during initial treatments
b) Explaining about the medications
c) Outlining about the expected follow up care after the treatment
d) Exploring with the hospice care

Question 40: A patient named Bill Bezos has been experiencing delirium. He is also suffering from marked confusions and hallucinations. Bill believes that the nurse is her daughter and he asks her if everyone at home is alright. The most appropriate reply for the nurse would be?

a) "I am not your child".
b) "Please stop dreaming bill".
c) "I am your nurse Mary Lisa"
d) "Yes, everyone is fine back home"

Question 41: Robin was provided with an adequate teaching in chemotherapy and Myelosuppression. He tries to demonstrate with his understanding. Which point is said to initiate his demonstration?
a) Myelosuppression occurs when there is an elevation in the white blood cell count.
b) Myelosuppression is a potential side effects to many cancer treatments.
c) Myelosuppression refers to the immune system reaction of the body to a particular medicine.
d) Myelosuppression is unintentional before blood transfusion

Question 42: William has been diagnosed with esophageal cancer. He suddenly reports having difficulty in swallowing and coughing. Which among the following will be considered more by the nurse?
a) Dry mouth
b) Acid reflex
c) Aspiration
d) Cavity

Question 43: What will be the duration of nadir to occur, after completing the chemotherapy treatment cycle?
a) 7- 10 days
b) 1- 3 weeks
c) 2- 5 weeks
d) 3 weeks

Question 44: Which among the following statements indicate the need for additional teaching regarding the coverage provided by the Family Medical Leave Act?
a) " It is difficult because my time off is unpaid "
b) " It helps me to take good care of my sister who is also a cancer patient "
c) " I know I'm eligible because I'm an American citizen"
d) " I can take up to 15 weeks of leave "

Question 45: A patient is at the dying stage due to lung cancer. The patient also feels dyspneic. What will the nurse do to make the patient feel less short of breath after finding that his bed is elevated to 45° and also noticed that he is receiving oxygen at 4L / min?
a) The nurse will turn the airflow of the pedestal fan towards the patient
b) The nurse tries to have a conversation with the patient
c) The nurse informs this to a physician
d) The nurse will make the patient lie flat on bed

Question 46: A patient has a platelet count of 15000/ mm^3. Which of following intervention should the nurse institute while attending the patient?
a) Using mouth swabs to complete oral care
b) Obtaining blood samples through large needles
c) Placing warm hot bags on the injected region
d) Providing massage to reduce the pain

Question 47: Which of the following conditions are included in Myeloablation for transplanting stem cell?
a) Retrograde surgical intervention
b) High dose chemotherapy
c) Growth analysis
d) Nutritional analysis

Question 48: Which among the following clearly denotes the 'purpose of a living will' , as taught by the nurse?
a) Acknowledgement of the risk and limiting the recommended therapies
b) Establishment of the patient's desire for care prior to a life threatening illness
c) Appointing surrogate to make medical decisions
d) Making final decision regarding treatment progression

Question 49: Michelle after entering a palliative care underwent a treatment for leukemia that included chemotherapy. The Absolute Neutrophil Count is 526/ mm^3, whereas her white blood cells close g is 5300/ mm^3. Michelle has higher risk for which among the following options?
a) Hypotension
b) Wheezing
c) Fracture
d) Infection

Question 50: While providing assistance in resolving patient's spiritual pain during end stage, what will be the prior intervention made by the nurse?
a) Acknowledge the legitimacy of the patient's pain
b) Encouraging patient to reduce focus on the issues
c) Encouraging reflection of random life events
d) Mobilizing patient's support system

Question 51: Robert, a 19 year old patient diagnosed with testicular cancer fears about his potency to conceive children as he will be receiving cisplatin and pelvic radiation. What will be suggested for Robert by the nurse?
a) Preserving the sperm before initiating the treatment

b) After the completion of the treatment, sildenafil is given to patient before engaging into sexual activity.
c) Sexual counseling throughout the treatment
d) Cryopreservation after completion of cisplatin treatment

Question 52: 5 mg of immediate release oxycodone is released 5 to 6 times daily when Mr.Smith receives 10mg of Sustained release Oxycodone for every 12 hours. Which of the following order has to be requested for the best adjustment in pain medication regimens?
a) 10 mg of immediate-release oxycodone every 12 hours
b) 30 mg of sustained-release oxycodone every 12 hours
c) 30 mg of immediate-release oxycodone every 6 hours
d) 10 mg of sustained-release oxycodone every 8 hours

Answer: b
Explanation: The duration of analgesia has to be decreased for the given opioid dose. When there is an improvement in analgesia, 25% opioid dosage is increased, for moderate and strong improvement 50% and 100% of the opioid dosage has to be improved respectively.

Question 53: Charles, a 21 year old cancer patient suddenly withdrew from college due to cancer resurrection. His family informs the nurse about his mood swings and refusal to meet his friends. What will be strategy achieved by the nurse initially?
a) Maintaining open communication
b) Re enrolling in college courses
c) Clinical trial participation
d) Recognizing self-destructive behavior

Question 54: Marcus with recurrent cancer is deteriorating due to his old age. His children are not sure of his wishes. Discussion with family and friends helps?
a) To divide the property of the patient equally

b) To agree with the hospital ethics teams
c) To find the available and appropriate option
d) To focus on family desire for the patient

Question 55: Occurrence of nausea is generally due to cancer or due to the treatment of cancer. Patient are taught with some basic self-care strategies that encourages patients to ?
a) High protein and potassium rich food
b) Consume sauces and gravies
c) Eat food that are cold at room temperature
d) Avoid brushing after nauseating

Question 56: Catherine, suffering from ovarian cancer develops severe nausea ending up vomiting in large volume of fluids. This causes abdominal pain and rigid palpation with diminishing bowel sounds due to little bowel movements. She is not feverish but feels difficulty in breathing. The most preferred diagnosis is:
a) Fecal impactions
b) Perforation of gastro intestinal tract
c) Colon Obstruction
d) Small Intestine Obstruction

Question 57: Michelle, a patient with breast cancer asks the nurse during counselling, "How long should I wait for my pregnancy after chemotherapy?". The nurse replies by saying,
a) No delay is necessary
b) Pregnancy will increase the chances of recurrence
c) You should wait at least one year
d) Infertility is said to be the permanent side effect of the therapy

Question 58: Robert, a patient with colon cancer underwent a bowel resection with colostomy. He suddenly experiences an abnormal finding on his third postoperative day. Which among the following matches his findings?
a) Slight stoma bleeding
b) Air in the ostomy appliances
c) Moist bright, pink stoma
d) A dull, grey stoma

Question 59: Aching and throbbing at a particular region is described as?
a) Referred pain
b) Somatic pain
c) Neuropathic pain
d) Pain in the internal organ

Question 60: Clara has been diagnosed with stage 3 cervical cancer. There are certain situations in which she may defer discussions about alteration in body image and sexual intimacy prior to the cancer treatment. Which among the following is likely to match the above reasons?
a) Expectation of experiencing minimal symptom for treatment
b) Concerned of being perceived as vain.
c) Depersonalization of the disease experience
d) Expectations of unrealistic outcomes

Question 61: A patient who is nearing death , was noticed with an audible gurgling during breathing by a nurse. How can the nurse explain the sound to the patient's family members visiting the patient?
a) "These are the side effects of his medications"

b) " This sound is normal for any patient at this stage"?
c) "Due to fluid accumulation, congestion in throat and lungs occur"
d) " He is at his end stage"

Question 62: Charles has been diagnosed with invasive ductal adenocarcinoma of pancreas. Upon diagnosis, the disease most likely:
a) Demonstrates the spread to liver
b) Displays the widespread fat globules
c) Remains without spreading to other body parts
d) Metastatic to Cartilage

Question 63: Harry, with small cell lung cancer has observed the following changes; increase of weight up to 4 pounds, headache and excessive thirst. These are generally the symptoms of?
a) Pericardial Tamponade
b) SIADH syndrome
c) Tumor lysis syndrome
d) Hemolytic Uremic Syndrome (HUS)

Question 64: William who has lung cancer reports of the following symptoms; A sudden acute pleura pain on his left side. He also exhibits dyspnea, Tachypnea, tachycardia, slight cough, and decreased sound in breathing over his left chest. These symptoms are due to?
a) Acute chest pain
b) Myocardial infarction
c) Lymphoma
d) Pneumothorax on left side

Question 65: What will be the primary nursing intervention of the patient who develops grade 3 peripheral neuropathy?
a) To teach about safe home environment
b) Monitor serum electrolytes
c) Recommend for increased narcotic analgesia
d) Obtain an order for corticosteroids

Question 66: The recently developed teaching booklet about immunotherapy was evaluated. It indicates that there is no increase in the group of patient's understanding about immunotherapy in the booklet. Which among the following has been considered as prominent principle?
a) Teaching is more effective when it responds to the need identified by the patient
b) Guideline for evaluation is provided depending on teacher's expectation
c) Verbal teaching increases the learning efficiency
d) The effectiveness of the learning is determined by the teaching methodology

Question 67: The primary purpose of providing multidisciplinary oncology care is to?
a) Improve patient's outcome
b) Improvise patient's communication
c) Meet the regulatory standards
d) Deliver cost effective services

Question 68: A gay man is at the dying stage because of leukemia. He asked the hospice not to allow his parents to meet him in his room as his parents didn't accept his lifestyle or his partner. What will be best action done by the nurse?
a) The nurse informs his parents about his unwillingness to meet them
b) The nurse can talk with the hospice
c) The nurse can request the patient to meet his parents

d) The nurse can ask his parents to leave a message as they are not allowed to meet him

Question 69: A cancer survivor is applying for a job interview. Which among the following should be done by the applicant during the initial interview?
a) The applicant has to contact the interviewer
b) The applicant has to explain about the personal qualifications for the job
c) The applicant should not provide details about his cancer treatment
d) The applicant has to provide medical information and current status

Question 70: Restlessness, insomnia, diarrhea, heart palpitations, and irritability are the reactions expressed by newly diagnosed cancer patient. Patient also gets nervous and worried and asks for some medication for nerves. What will be the best response from the nurse?
a) Informs the patient about the initiation of treatment
b) Ask the patient to explain his feelings further
c) Assure that the reason is due to cancer diagnosis
d) Instructs the patient to ask for a sedative from the physician.

Question 71: Who has a higher risk of skin breakdown?
a) A patient with decreased sensory perception.
b) Higher mobilized patient
c) A patient with decreased serum albumin level
d) A patient with hyperpigmentation

Question 72: The most effective treatment for the severe pain that is associated with the post herpetic neuropathy is?

a) Amitriptyline
b) Propoxyphene
c) Extra strength acetaminophen
d) Dihydromorphinone

Question 73: Which of the following intervention is suggested to the patient who has dry desquamation?
a) Moisturizing skin cream
b) Silver sulphadiazine
c) Aloe Vera dressing
d) Hydrogel dressing

Question 74: Weight loss, abdominal pain and diarrhea are some of the symptoms reported by Harry who is 70 years old. He also reported that these symptoms often interrupts his sleep. Harry's brother was recently diagnosed for prostate cancer. What will the nurse suspect?
a) Neurofibromatosis
b) Carcinoid syndrome
c) Spastic colon
d) Klinefelter syndrome

Question 75: Temozolomide are used for administering certain brain cancer. What will be nurse advice to patient who is about to begin temozolomide medication?
a) Weekly monitoring the amount of protein in urine is necessary
b) Diarrhea is the common side effects
c) Neutropenia occurs after 22 to 28 days of completion
d) Uncommon side effects are nausea and vomiting

Question 76: A patient who is at the dying state experiences delirium. Medication that can manage this symptom will be?
a) Aprepitant
b) Paracetamol

c) Haloperidol
d) Cetirizine

Question 77: Richard reports of certain symptoms after receiving a high dose of external beam radiation for lung cancer 8 weeks ago. This symptoms include development of dyspnea and non productive cough. In the area of his previous radiation treatment, a chest x-ray shows open ground glass opacification. Which among the following is the result of the above symptoms?
a) Bilateral atelectasis
b) Cardiac tamponade
c) Increased libidos
d) Radiation pneumonitis

Question 78: Which among the following measures provides relief for the patient who has had persistent nausea and vomiting despite of receiving medication for controlling the symptoms?
a) By taking a deep breath and having control of swallowing manners
b) By laying flat on the floor
c) By avoiding dinner
d) By in taking large volume of fluid

Question 79: Persistent fever and chills has been reported by a patient receiving interleukin 2 with neutrophils count of 1500/mm^3. What is the representation of these symptoms?
a) Drug induced reaction
b) Viral infection
c) Septic shock
d) Tumor lysis syndrome

Question 80: Clara has a history of ovarian cancer suddenly reports feeling full after eating small quantity and also experiences an increase in weight. She has noticed an increase of 10 pounds within a week and also states that she is eating less. What will the nurse instruct Clara?
a) Call when is there is an increase in swelling of ankle.
b) Report if there is an increase in weight
c) Eat small and frequent meals
d) Visit the clinic

Question 81: Which of the following disease can be cured by allogeneic stem cell transplant?
a) Acute lymphoblastic leukemia
b) Germ cell tumors
c) Lymphoma
d) Breast Cancer

Question 82: The patient has sudden dyspnea, wheezing, hypotension, throat and face swelling during the administration of chemotherapeutic agent intravenously. What will be the initial action of the nurse?
a) To increase administering epinephrine
b) To discontinue the administering of chemotherapeutic agent
c) To stop administering oxygen
d) To decrease antihistamine

Question 83: Among the following option, which is the best mediation to increase the patient's adherence for taking oral chemotherapy at home?
a) It will be easier to monitor the patient regarding the side effects
b) In order to make the patient feel convenient about taking a double dose in case if the patient missed the medication

c) It will be easier for the patient to take up the refill when the supply runs out during the next appointment
d) In order make the patient take over the counter medicine for nausea

Question 84: Which among the following technique supports the healthy communication pattern between the patient and nurse?
a) Feedbacks has to be obtained regarding the preferences and experiences
b) Physical distance has to be established between the parties
c) After providing all the information, the questions has to be limited.
d) The objective and factual information has to be provided regarding the treatment plan

Question 85: Radiation therapy is given to the patient with a tumor on the floor of the mouth. What advice is given to the patient?
a) Consume only less fluid everyday
b) Avoid using less spices
c) Avoid using topical anesthetic
d) Avoid consuming alcohol

Question 86: Merlin, a cancer patient has lost four pounds since the beginning of her Chemotherapy-treatment. What will be first reaction of the nurse after finding it during her home visit?
a) Arrange for meals on the wheels service
b) Investigates the reason for weight loss
c) Asks Merlin to consult physician
d) Suggests high-protein and high calorie-food

Question 87: A cancer patient reports of following symptoms; appearance of white lesions on the tongue and inside of her cheeks, the tissues is irritated painful with slight bleeding. Which among the following is the best treatment?
a) Mouth wash with lemon swabs
b) Ampicillin
c) Nystatin an antifungal medication for oral suppression
d) Caphosol

Question 88: Mortality rate can be reduced by using acetyl salicylic acid for which of the following cancer types?
a) Malignant neoplasm of testis
b) Cervical
c) Leukemia
d) Gastrointestinal

Question 89: Michele is using fentanyl patches to control her pain caused due to ovarian cancer. She reports the nurse regarding the following symptoms; Difficulty in urinating and able to pass only small amount of urine. Bladder is not distended and has bilateral pain in the flank areas. Recent blood test reports shows slight hyperkalemia and is afebrile. These symptoms are due to?
a) Cervical cancer
b) Infection in bladder
c) Side effects caused by the intake of opioids
d) Obstruction in upper urinary tract

Question 90: While discussing the ethical principles regarding the side effects of chemotherapy to a staff, the nurse tries to put forth her point saying that positive effects should bring more good effects than the negative effects bringing bad. Which of the following ethical principle is this related?
a) Autonomy
b) Beneficence

c) Justice
d) Non harming or inflicting least harm.

Question 91: There is a significant increase in the risk of developing a breast cancer. Which among the following people has a higher chance of risk?
a) First pregnancy at age of 31
b) Menopause at the age of 53
c) Menarche at age 13
d) Mother diagnosed before 60 years of age

Question 92: Among the following, who has increased risk of developing a graft-versus-host disease?
a) A 42-years- old patient received a syngeneic hematopoietic stem cell transplant
b) A 25-years-old patient received a tandem autologous stem cell transplant
c) A 30-years- old patient received an autologous hematopoietic stem cells transfer
d) A 60-years-old patient received an allogeneic transplant from a unrelated donor.

Question 93: Michelle, a patient has a negative result for BRCA mutation but her sister Rosie has a positive result. What kind of emotion does Michelle exhibit when she says with tears," I was always the troublesome kid"?
a) Transmitter guilt
b) Survivor Guilt
c) Reactive Depression
d) Siblings rivalry

Question 94: A newly diagnosed patient enquires the nurse about all the tests for clinical staging as suggested by doctor. Which among the following will be the answer given by nurse according to her knowledge regarding staging?
a) Predicts response to treatment
b) Evaluates the extend of local and potential metastatic disease
c) Compares the result across population
d) Assess usual spreading pattern of cancer

Question 95: The policy and procedure for chemotherapy administration has been reviewed by nurse's manager. In what ways can the ASCO/ ONS Chemotherapy Administration for Safety Standards assist in this process?
a) It helps in providing description for the oncology nurse jobs
b) The data collection tool regarding the quality improvement are provided
c) It provides idea about the professional responsibility of the oncology nurses in chemotherapy administration.
d) The required educational classes for the oncology nurses are being listed

Question 96: Which of the following cancer type should be screened by 25 year old Michelle with BRCA1 mutation, who also underwent Bilateral Preventative Mastectomies for Breast Cancer?
a) Breast Cancer
b) Ovarian Cancer
c) Lymphatic Cancer
d) Brain Cancer

Question 97: William is experiencing uncontrolled pain due to bone metastasis. The nurse, the patient and the palliative care are reviewing the plan of care. The above scenario is an example of?
a) Advising
b) Collaboration

c) Advising
d) Criticize

Question 98: For managing nausea and Vomiting at the end of the life, which of the following complimentary is most likely to be effective?
a) Acupuncture
b) Music therapy
c) Massage
d) Walking

Question 99: What type of cancer can be prevented when oral contraceptive pills are consumed for more than 5 years?
a) Breast cancer
b) Ovarian cancer
c) Lung cancer
d) Endometrial cancer

Question 100: Among the following, which one causes more blisters or is a vesicant?
a) Dactinomycin
b) Topotecan
c) Melphalan
d) Dalcabazine

Question 101: A patient with renal carcinoma has been administered with sunitinib. Patient reports of burning sensation, tingling and redness in the palm and foot while receiving sunitinib. Which among the following is the result of the above symptoms?
a) Palmar plantar erythrodysesthesia
b) Darkened patches and spots on skin
c) Acneiform rash
d) Erythema multiform major

Question 102: Rihanna has been diagnosed with breast cancer. She has been receiving radiation therapy. She reports to her nurse over her decreased libidos. What will be the appropriate nursing interventions?
a) Gives instructions about the vaginal dilators
b) Explores patient's feeling regarding sexular activity
c) Reassures the patient that it will return
d) Recommend look good feel better programs

Question 103: William requires chronic platelet transfusions may develop antibodies and require further products to be:
a) Delayed
b) Low body mass index
c) Leukoreduced
d) Reduced volume

Question 104: Which among the following should the nurse focus while considering rehabilitation principle in a cancer patient?
a) Develop group goals
b) Encouraging more rest periods
c) Emphasize capabilities
d) Focusing more on disabilities

Question 105: Janet is newly diagnosed with cancer so she has quit her job and other social activity. What will be the nurse's response to Janet?
a) By encouraging her that she will be able to join after treatment
b) By saying that her friends would be proud of Janet being a brave overcoming cancer
c) By asking about the activity she enjoyed the most before starting treatment
d) By asking her to focus on her cancer

Question 106: A Fluorouracil based chemotherapy combination has been administered to Ron, who has been employed as a landscaper. Which among the following symptom is most likely to occur?
a) Gouty arthritis
b) Photosensitivity
c) Pulmonary toxicity
d) Accumulation of fluid in lower limbs

Question 107:   Continuous Quality Improvement, or CQI, is a management philosophy that organizations use to reduce waste, increase efficiency, and increase internal (meaning, employees) and external (meaning, customer) satisfaction. Which among the following is the core concept of CQI?
a) Institute organizational transparency
b) Problems relate to processes and variations in process lead to variations in results
c) Change emanates from the top
d) Systemic process improvement to be successful

Question 108: Darbepoetin Alfa has been administered for the patient with advanced stage of breast cancer. Which among the following are the risk associated according to patient's understanding?
a) Risk are only for those who have large tumors
b) With each injection the risk of bleeding and infections get doubled.
c) Improvement in anemia and the disease may progress
d) Improvement of anemia causing less risk

Question 109: What is considered as the most important factor for self-determined closure of life?
a) Stopping the treatment
b) Honoring wishes of patient regarding end of life care
c) Proceeding with advanced medication

d) Discharging the patient

Question 110: A patient who has been enrolled in clinical trials has made an informed decision. Which among the following suitably match his informed decision?
a) Though there is no positive response from family, patient believes the process
b) The physician has explained all these to my family
c) Physician wouldn't have suggested if it was not suitable.
d) Gained knowledge from cancer blog and came to know about its survival rate

Question 111: The most likely cause of palmar plantar erythrodysesthesia is?
a) Rupture of capillaries due to pressure and friction
b) Arranging for an occupational therapy
c) Over exposure of fast growing skin cells
d) Decreased circulation after infusion

Question 112: Breast cancer survivor suddenly weeps to a nurse saying that she didn't expect that lymphedema would happen to her. How will the nurse react the patient?
a) By taking a recent history to identify the occurrence of lymphedema
b) By teaching the prevention methods of lymphedema recurrence
c) By allowing the patient to express her feelings
d) By assuring the quick recovery of lymphedema

Question 113: Mark who has colon mesothelioma has been scheduled for chemotherapy which is to be administered in the peritoneal space. Which is the type of device through which Mark attends his chemotherapy?
a) Large diameter silicon port implantation
b) Arterial Catheter
c) Intraventricular catheter reservoir (Ommaya reservoir)

d) Insertion of central catheter peripherally

Question 114: What will be the choice of treatment for the patient with stage 1 non-small cell lung cancer with impaired pulmonary functions?
a) Removal of Lung (pneumactomy) (lobectomy)
b) Platinum based chemotherapy
c) Removal of lobe of an organ
d) External beam radiation

Question 115: When the adult children of the patient who passed away approaches the nurse expressing the feelings, then the nurse can provide support to the family by?
a) Encouraging discussion with Physician
b) Validating the necessity of counseling for these feelings
c) Validating these as normal feelings of grief
d) Encouraging a family conference

Question 116: A nurse is working with a patient with terminal illness. Which among the following statement seems to be helpful for her in assisting her patient to reframe hope?
a) "What appears to be more important to you?"
b) "We are always there to help you"
c) "You are still left with more time, don't worry"
d) "Have faith in God, he will save you"

Question 117: Oral mucositis is caused by?
a) Amoxicillin
b) Fluorouracil
c) Interleukin 2
d) Paracetamol

Question 118: What is the long term complication for the patient who is receiving hormonal therapy for prostate cancer?
a) Adverse skeletal events
b) Ulcers

c) Lymphedema
d) Cardiac dysfunction

Question 119: What type of chemotherapy induced nausea does the patient experience after four days of chemotherapy?
a) Prolonged
b) Refractory
c) Acute
d) Delayed

Question 120: A nurse has been assigned to take care of 5 patients. She provides documentation and assessment for only 4 patients as she had misread the entire agreement. The legal principle that applies to this situation is?
a) Breach of duty
b) Dereliction of duty
c) Testimonial proof
d) Non harming

Question 121: Harry, Colon cancer survivor wishes to change his job. But he fears that he won't be able to receive his insurance due to his cancer history. What will the nurse advice?
a) Provides contact of National Coalition of cancer survivorship.
b) Inform him about the Americans with Disabilities Act of 1990
c) Refer him to a support group
d) Encourages him to speak with a lawyer

Question 122: When a nurse has the ability to recognize and respect difference in beliefs, values and lifestyle, which among the following will the nurse try to demonstrate?
a) Non maleficence
b) Protective buffering
c) Cultural competence
d) Presentation

Question 123: Clara, a 20 year old childhood brain cancer survivor is complaining about her sudden weight gain, weakness in muscles, dysmenorrhea and depression. At the age of 5, she underwent radiation therapy and surgery as treatment for cancer. The above symptoms are the later effects of?
a) Cardiomyopathy
b) Hypothyroidism
c) Resurgence of Cancer
d) Lack of healthy red blood cells

Question 124: Which among the following will be the major side effects received by the patient due to the intake of irinotecan?
a) Diarrhea
b) Constriction of pupil of eye
c) Patchy hair loss
d) Expelling stomach content out of mouth forcefully

Question 125: The following are the symptoms of a patient suffering from stage IV Lung Cancer; Difficulty in differentiating between anginal pain (progressive dyspnea), facial swelling; swelling of neck, arms,hands and thorax due to the fluid from the tissue; Distended jugular,temporal and arm veins; disturbance in vision; headache and disorientation (altered mental status). The diagnosis for the above symptoms are:
a) Lung embolism
b) Syndrome for Inappropriate secretion of Anti-Diuretic Hormone (SIADH)
c) Superior Vena Cava Syndrome (SVCS)
d) Compression of Spinal Cord

Question 126: The role of proto oncogene is to ?
a) Promote cell division
b) Stimulate angiogenesis
c) Causes programmed cell death
d) Promote cell division

Question 127: The need for descending colostomy has been discussed with John who has Colorectal cancer. What will be the position of stoma?
a) Right lower quadrant
b) Left upper quadrant
c) Left lower quadrant
d) Just below the waistline

Question 128: Patient who has been undergoing treatment for cancer fails to respond to the treatment. When this has been informed to the patient, what will be the initial nursing interventions?
a) Asking family members to provide verbal support
b) Reviewing the treatment possibilities as referred by the physician
c) Providing time for self processing by the patient
d) Asks the patient to share the feelings after hearing the news

Question 129: Michelle has metastatic breast cancer. She experiences pain at the site of metastasis during the initiation of tamoxifen. Which among the following clearly explains the pain?
a) A common temporary reaction to the initiation therapy
b) Due to progression of disease
c) A Psychosomatic reaction due to the diagnosis of metastasis
d) Due to improper sleeping position

Question 130: In order to reduce anxiety which among the following is suggested?
a) Mindfulness-based stress reduction
b) Meditation
c) Hyperbaric oxygen therapy
d) Allopathy

Question 131: Watson expresses his willingness to return back to work after treatment. But sometimes he reports of feeling fatigue. Which among the following is considered as the suitable step for his problem?
a) Having a break for a 2 years before commencing work schedule
b) Asking the family member to work and continue with household chores.
c) Avoiding discussion with his co-workers who are sick
d) Discussing with his officials regarding flexible work time.

Question 132: What action will the nurse take if the family members of the dying patient disagree on placing the feeding tube?
a) Meets the family to discuss the goals of care
b) Communicates with the social workers to begin the process
c) Explains that only the management can make decisions
d) Encourages the family to go through similar cases

Question 133: A patient is receiving Fluorouracil and leucovorin for an unresectable T2 N2 M1 adenocarcinoma of the colon. Which among the following is considered as the goal for this treatment?
a) Control in cancer growth
b) Increase in cellular contact inhibition
c) Radio sensitivity promotion
d) Promotion of cellular transformation

Question 134: A patient diagnosed with breast cancer was given a dose of IV doxorubicin an anthracycline DNA-binding agent. Soon the patient was observed to be suffering from symptoms like swelling, redness, itching and vesicles at IV insertion site. The course of action that the nurse should follow after discontinuing the medication is:
a) The nurse should apply some ice and administer dexrazoxane.
b) The nurse should apply some heat and administer dexrazoxane.

c) The nurse should apply some heat and administer dimethyl sulfoxide.
d) The nurse should apply some ice and administer dimethyl sulfoxide.

Question 135: A patient's temperature is 39*C and she has tachypnea, tachycardia and leukocytosis (20,000/mm3).She is an immunocompromised patient and she has developed a systematic infection. The infection would be classified as:
a) Bacteremia.
b) Multi organ disinfection syndrome
c) Systemic inflammatory response syndrome.
d) None of the above.

Question 136: During her childhood, Rosie has received Carmustine. Now, being a 24 year old adult she reports of persistent cough and shortness in breath. Which of the following has high risk of development?
a) Allergic reaction to the fungus
b) Accumulation of pus in pleural space
c) Lung embolism
d) Pulmonary Fibrosis

Question 137: List the two types of cancer for which hormone therapy is effective?
a) Breast and prostate
b) Leukemia and breast
c) Liver and prostate
d) Liver and lymphoma

Question 138: Which of the following medications requires mandatory enrollment in a program to ensure teaching about risks to a fetus is provided?
a) Sorafenib
b) Everolimus
c) Capecitabine

d) Lenalidomide

Question 139: The required premedication causes drowsiness. The nurse informs the patient about the drowsiness that occurs due to medication. Therefore the patient request the nurse for delaying the treatment so that patient performs the prayer during sunset. The nurse should first
a) Assess to determine if a delay is permissible
b) Informing the patient that the treatment can't be delayed
c) Require that a waiver be signed to delay treatment
d) Delay the treatment for 24 hours

Question 140: In order to determine acute changes in nutritional status and also to monitor the dietary status of patient with cachexia, test are generally taken. Which of the following is most commonly monitored ?
a) Albumin and Globulin
b) Albumin
c) Transferrin
d) Prealbumin

Question 141: At what age prostate specific antigen blood test has to be taken in order to reduce average risk according to American Cancer society Guidelines?
a) 30
b) 40
c) 20
d) 50

Question 142: After hematopoietic stem cell transplant, Robert was taught about the discharge medication. Which among the following explains the purpose of tacrolimus?
a) It prevents Nausea and vomiting sensation
b) It prevents graft-versus-host disease
c) It helps to prevent fungal pneumonia
d) It avoids sinusoidal obstruction syndrome

Question 143: Richard has completed treatment for neck and head cancer. He is at high risk for which secondary malignancy?
a) Glioblastoma multiforme
b) Lung cancer
c) Kidney cancer
d) Bile duct cancer

Question 144: What type of nausea does the patient receive after 48 hours of chemotherapy?
a) Short term
b) Breakthrough
c) Delayed
d) Somatic

Question 145: What combines with a mouse to form a cosmetic monoclonal antibody?
a) cow antibody
b) Human antibody
c) Pig antibody
d) Plant antibody

Question 146: Ronnie Reacts by displaying maladaptive response for the diagnosis of cancer. This indicates that Ronnie is?
a) Focusing to live in the present moment
b) Feeling abandoned by God
c) Fighting the treatment for his children

d) Lowering his concentration on treatment

Question 147: Which of the following cancer is associated with a patient exposed to radon for a longer duration?
a) Lung Cancer
b) Breast Cancer
c) Colorectal / Bowel Cancer
d) Bladder Cancer

Question 148: A patient with lymphoma feels weak while ambulating and dribbling urine and also experience numbness in feet. Which among the following will be the initial suspect by the nurse?
a) Endocrine disruptor
b) Type 1 diabetes
c) Spinal cord compression
d) Peripheral neuritis

Question 149: Which among the following is an example for adaptive or specific immunity?
a) Cell mediated response
b) Acute phase protein production
c) Large lymphocyte production
d) Inflammatory response

Question 150: A patient is treated with posaconazole. Which of the following side effects should be informed to the patient regarding the treatment?
a) Bone marrow aplasia
b) Anemia
c) Pancreatitis
d) Torsades de Pointes

Question 151: Thrombocytopenia is referred as the decrease in the number of circulating platelets below $100,000/mm^3$. What has to be taught to the patient to avoid the risk due to thrombocytopenia?
a) Using soft bristled toothbrush
b) Walking barefoot
c) High fiber food consumption
d) Having a haircut

Question 152: To whom is the nurse responsible to according to ANA code of ethics?
a) Patient
b) Herself
c) Medical Council
d) Physician

Question 153: In what ways does the cancer cell differ from the ordinary cells?
a) Ordinary cells generally reside in new areas
b) Ordinary cells doesn't allow contact with the other cells
c) Cancer cells migrate to the neighboring locations and tissues
d) Cancer cells divide only when the older cells are destroyed

Question 154: A patient receiving a high dosage of methotrexate is administered with intravenous fluid containing sodium bicarbonate. This is done to:
a) Eliminate the leucovorin rescue needs
b) Maintain alkaline urine
c) Reduce sensitivity to reaction
d) Protect against Vomiting

Question 155: Name the governmental organization which is responsible for the protection of human subjects and states that when performing studies involving human beings, the researcher must first obtain informed consent, in an easily understandable manner?
a) CDC
b) PAHO
c) FDA
d) WHO

Question 156: A patient with permanent colostomy expresses concern of having sexual intercourse. What will the nurse recommend initially?
a) Discuss with the therapist before having a sexual intercourse
b) Track bowel habits to schedule sexual intercourse
c) Replace ostomy appliance just before the sexual intercourse
d) Have food before engaging in sexual intercourse

Question 157: A Lymphedema patient was reported using reflexology for the affected arm who was seen in the outpatient clinic. What will the nurse enquire?
a) Lymphedema will subside over time
b) This method has a promising cure in clinical trials
c) Can u provide me with more information on this technique?
d) Recommending to use compression sleeve

Question 158: Louis receives total body irradiation for hematopoietic stem cell transplant. After one year he reports dullness in vision and ocular sensitivity. What is said to be the cause of above symptoms?
a) Cataract
b) Loss of vision
c) Optic neuritis
d) Crossed eye

Question 159: Within a week of chemotherapy a patient with acute lymphoid leukemia experience the following symptoms; Hyperkalemia, Hyperphosphatemia and Hypocalcemia. The above symptoms indicate?
a) Tumor Lysis Syndrome
b) Consumptive coagulopathy
c) Septic shock
d) Hyponatremia and hypo-osmolality

Question 160: In order to reduce the noise rattled breathing for a dying patient which of the following non pharmacological interventions is suitable?
a) Increasing the morphine infusion rate
b) Relocating/Repositioning to clear secretion
c) Executing nasopharyngeal suctions
d) Humidifying oxygen

Answers & Explanation

Answers with Explanation

Question 1:
Answer: a
Explanation: According to the American Cancer Society, digital rectal examination and prostate specific antigen testing are considered to be made as the necessary test that has to be taken beginning at the age of 45 for men in concern with the high risk of prostate cancer.

Question 2:
Answer:d
Explanation: Whenever the hazardous medication are realized into the environment due to any spill, face shield will provide proper protection from any sudden splash causing damage to the eyes and face while cleaning the spill.

Question 3:
Answer: b
Explanation: Naproxen is a nonsteroidal anti-inflammatory drug used to treat pain. Cytoprotection is a process by which the chemical compounds provide protection to the cells from the damage created by harmful agents. It is advisable to consult a physician regarding the cytoprotectants.

Question 4:
Answer: a
Explanation: Anaphase is the shortest phase of mitosis. In anaphase, the sister chromatids are pulled apart to opposite ends of the cell.

Question 5:
Answer: c
Explanation: Increased intracranial pressure shows symptoms such as restlessness and confusion.

Question 6:
Answer: c
Explanation: An unconscious process refers to sadness that is associated with a shock or sudden unhappy news. Generally anticipatory grief is associated with an unconscious process.

Question 7
Answer: d
Explanation: Anticipatory nausea can be prevented by integrative or complimentary therapy. These generally include Acupuncture, massage, music therapy etc.

Question 8:
Answer: d
Explanation: Reiki is a form of alternative medicine called energy healing. Reiki practitioners use a technique called palm healing or hands-on healing through which a "universal energy" is said to be transferred through the palms of the practitioner to the patient in order to encourage emotional or physical healing. It would be appropriate for the patient with low platelet count.

Question 9:
Answer: b
Explanation: Birth control pills and the barrier methods are suggested by the physician before initiating chemotherapy

Question 10:
Answer: a
Explanation: Myelosuppression or bone marrow depression generally occurs for the patient who receives chemotherapy and also radiation treatment.

Question 11:
Answer: a

Explanation: It is better to assist William with scheduled defecation every day and about half an hour after every meal. This is because it helps to stimulate the gastro colic reflex that propels the fecal matter through colon. This can be sometimes stimulated by any stimulus but the usage has to be minimized during the progressive days. William has to maintain a proper record about his stool evacuation and its consistency.

Question 12:
Answer: c
Explanation: While using alkylating agent the risk for having secondary leukemia increases for Michelle. Here the alkylating agent is cyclophosphamide.

Question 13:
Answer: b
Explanation: Survivorship care plan has the following benefits to the patient: It shall provide complete information regarding the treatment received, the long term effects and the healthy choice of lifestyle and screenings throughout their life term.

Question 14
Answer: b
Explanation: Some of the prescribed drugs can affect the platelet function and must be reviewed. This is because sometimes these symptoms with normal platelet count may suggest another cause.

Question 15:
Answer: b
Explanation: Bone is said to be the frequent site for occurrence of metastasis whereas Liver and Lung experiences rare spread of metastatic effect.

Question 16:
Answer: c

Explanation: An individual who has cancer shows true positive result during the cancer screening. There are no considerations for the individual with other characteristics.

Question 17
Answer: b
Explanation: When a nurse develops an educational program, the key point to be noted is to assess learning requirements. This is the categorized as the first step in determining educational objectives, selecting educational methods, and later formulates criteria for evaluation.

Question 18:
Answer: c
Explanation: Pain is generally considered as punishment therefore the nurse helps in confronting the family about this opinion and brings positive mind.

Question 19:
Answer: b
Explanation: Complicated grief is generally unresolved or it can take a long duration to resolve. This is caused due to the loss of a closest people or with whom they are living with. Therefore it better to stay away from having conversation about the descendant.

Question 20:
Answer: d
Explanation: Loperamide is a medication used to decrease the frequency of diarrhea. It is often used for this purpose in, inflammatory bowel disease, and short bowel syndrome. It is not recommended for those with blood in the stool, mucus in the stool or fevers.

Question 21:
Answer: b

Explanation: Alkylating agent generally binds with the DNA strand, breaks the DNA helix strand and interferes with DNA replication. It also prevents the occurrence of cell division.

Question 22:
Answer: b
Explanation: Lymphatic cancer rates are up to 5% for the females who underwent sentinel lymph node procedure and rates are from 10 to 30% for females after axillary lymph node dissection.

Question 23
Answer: a
Explanation: Tumor invades into the vertebrae causing collapse on the spinal cord that results in impending spinal cord compression. High risk for compression is generally for the patients with prostate cancer. Dull back pain is known to be the earlier symptom of spinal cord compression.

Question 24:
Answer: c
Explanation: The Buddhists leave the body undisturbed for a long period of time because they believe that a soul needs some time to leave the body and be at peace. The Buddhists believe in multiple lifetimes like the Hindus and they also believe that the actions of their past lives might affect their present one. They call this as karma.

Question 25
Answer: b
Explanation: In order to maintain blood pressure and tissue perfusion, the antibiotic therapy generally based on the site of infection and most likely a causative pathogen.

Question 26
Answer: b

Explanation: Development of unexpanded lung or trapped lung is the cause of repeated thoracentesis.

Question 27:
Answer: d
Explanation: Patients who are not considered for cytotoxic chemotherapy are administered with Gemtuzumab ozogamicin usually above 60 years of age.

Question 28:
Answer: c
Explanation: Dimethicone is used as a moisturizer to treat or prevent dry, rough, scaly, itchy skin and minor skin irritations such as skin burns from radiation therapy. These are substances that soften and moisturize the skin and decrease itching and flaking.

Question 29:
Answer: a
Explanation: The common symptom of oral mucositis is pain. Other symptoms include Red, shiny or swollen mouth and gums, Blood in the mouth, Sores in the mouth or on the gums or tongue, Soreness or pain in the mouth or throat, Difficulty swallowing or talking.

Question 30
Answer: a
Explanation: Cancer surgery generally removes the tumor and the nearby tissue during an operation. It is one among the oldest treatment but it is still effective.

Question 31:
Answer: c

Explanation: Microscopic examination of the cell is required by the histologic headings in order to explain their resemblance as normal cells. These cells usually grow and spread at a normal rate. But the cells which are undifferentiated tend to be more aggressive and they spread more easily. They also grow rapidly. These cells are known as tumor cells. Every tumor cell has it's own level, higher the grade the more aggressive it becomes.

Question 32
Answer: a
Explanation: Condition of spinal cord compression occurs as tumors invade epidural space of spinal cord. Symptoms include back pain, muscle loss, reduced bladder function and vertebral tiredness. Fast growing tumor are treated with surgery and others with radiation.

Question 33:
Answer: b
Explanation: Oligodendroglia create myelin sheaths for CNS axons, paralleling the function of Schwann cells in the peripheral nervous system. It generally develops and maintains the Myelin sheath.

Question 34
Answer: a
Explanation: By using alcohol and smokeless tobacco together can cause Laryngeal cancer. It increases the risk of development up to to 50%.

Question 35
Answer: a
Explanation: When a patient is scheduled to receive Oxaliplatin, intake of ice chips and cold foods has to be avoided along with the fluids.

Question 36:
Answer: c

Explanation: Smoking is responsible for almost 90% of the total cases of lung cancer. Smoking is also responsible for various other types of cancer. All cancer patients are advised to discontinue the use of tobacco and they are also asked to quit smoking.

Question 37:
Answer: a
Explanation: Greater risk for sexual difficulties are more likely to be experienced by the patients who were having marital issue in their relationship before the diagnosis of cancer.

Question 38:
Answer: a
Explanation: Dexamethasone is used as it prevents fluid retention. It is also used to reduce inflammation and suppress (lower) the body's immune response. It is used with other drugs to treat the following types of cancer: Leukemia. Lymphoma.

Question 39
Answer: c
Explanation: By providing the patient with long term follow up care after treatment is the main aim of cancer survivorship plan. Appropriate schedule for screening, early and late effects of the treatments, description of the therapies are some of the other information included in the cancer survivorship plan.

Question 40:
Answer:c
Explanation: It would be very helpful for the patient if the nurse tries to orient him by clarifying his name. Delirium is very common for the patients who are at the end of their life.

Question 41:
Answer: b

Explanation: The response of the immune system is decreased by causing neutropenia, anemia and thrombocytopenia during chemotherapy. This is generally referred as Myelosuppression. Therefore it is said to be the potential side effect of many cancer types.

Question 42:
Answer:c
Explanation: High risk of obstructive dysphagia in esophageal cancer generally leads to Aspiration.

Question 43:
Answer: a
Explanation: After completing the complete chemotherapy cycle, nadir occurs within 7- 10 days after chemotherapy.

Question 44:
Answer: c
Explanation: The Family and Medical Leave Act of 1993 is a United States labor law requiring covered employers to provide employees with job-protected and unpaid leave for qualified medical and family reasons. It provides unpaid leave to care for the family member who is seriously affected due to cancer.

Question 45:
Answer: a
Explanation: By directing the fan towards the patient, the patient shall overcome the fear of feeling short of breath. By making the patient lie flat on bed doesn't increase the airflow. Usually 2 to 4L/min oxygen is administered to the patient. By altering the fluid intake does not affect dyspnea as the breathlessness is associated with lung cancer.

Question 46
Answer: a

Explanation: Sponges and bristle less toothbrush are used for the patient who has platelets counts less than 20,000/ mm³. Therefore it is advised to complete the oral care with mouth swabs.

Question 47:
Answer: b
Explanation: Myeloablation refers to total body irradiation that prevents autologous hematologic recovery. By administering high dosage of chemotherapy, residual disease can be eliminated prior to hematopoietic stem cell transplant.

Question 48:
Answer: b
Explanation: In case of any terminal illness, the determination of care that a patient is willing to receive is based on the patient's willingness to live.

Question 49:

Answer: b
Explanation: If the Absolute Neutrophil Count (ANC) falls below 1000mm³, then there is a chance of increase in risk rapidly. The normal neutrophil count of an adult is 1800 to 7700 mm³. Neutropenia occurs if the ANC decreases. Neutropenia is the severe complication in chemotherapy and other diseases such as leukemia. If a patient has both neutropenia and fever then the patient is prone to an infection that becomes life threatening.

Question 50:
Answer: a
Explanation: Patients from spiritual and cultural background tend to cause spiritual distress. Encourage verbalization and use family venogram to draw out relationships, fears, hopes and unfinished business will be considered as best acknowledgement of client's spiritual pain.

Question 51
Answer: a
Explanation: Sperm banking is recommended before initiating the treatment with cisplatin and pelvic radiation. This is because chemotherapy with cisplatin and alkylating agents can cause permanent infertility (Azoospermia). For future paternity Robert is suggested with sperm banking.

Question 52
Answer: b
Explanation: The duration of analgesia has to be decreased for the given opioid dose. When there is an improvement in analgesia, 25% opioid dosage is increased, for moderate and strong improvement 50% and 100% of the opioid dosage has to be improved respectively.

Question 53
Answer: a
Explanation: Only when Charles starts to communicate with his family and friends, he shall be able to feel the support and value for his feeling through his communication so that he can be little better.

Question 54
Answer: d
Explanation: A proper communication between the nurse and the family members ensures to gain more information on Marcus's last wishes.

Question 55
Answer: c
Explanation: In addition to pharmacological management, patient are given self-care treatments such as eating food that are cold at room temperature as the aroma of hot food increases nausea.

Question 56

Answer: d
Explanation: These are consistent symptoms of small intestine obstruction. Bowel obstruction occurs due to sudden and frequent nausea and vomiting in large volumes. Dexamethasone can relieve few symptoms as it reduces inflammation and swelling and also provides relief to nausea.

Question 57:
Answer: c
Explanation: There is no decrease in the women who gets pregnant after chemotherapy. Therefore, Michelle is recommended to wait one to five years following cessation of all treatment.

Question 58
Answer: d
Explanation: A moist reddish pink is said to be the normal condition of healthy stoma. Robert experiences a dull grey stoma due to lack of blood flow, ischemia or necrosis. In this case Robert has to immediately report to a physician.

Question 59:
Answer: b
Explanation: Somatic pain occurs when pain receptors in tissues (including the skin, muscles, skeleton, joints, and connective tissues) are activated. Typically, stimuli such as force, temperature, vibration, or swelling activate these receptors.

Question 60:
Answer: b
Explanation: Sometimes while having a discussion with her partner about sexuality Clara seems to feel like being in vain, as she feels that the discussion seems to inappropriate and can embarrass when compared to the seriousness of her treatment.

Question 61:
Answer: c

Explanation: This condition has to be explained by the nurse in a non-frightening terms. The nurse has to avoid conveying it negatively such as stating about his end stage and also about the side effects. The nurse should not give any false hope saying that the condition is normal during this stage. If the gurgling sound is distressing to the family or if it's severe then medications can be given.

Question 62
Answer: a
Explanation: Invasive ductal carcinoma (IDC), sometimes called infiltrating ductal carcinoma, is the most common type of breast cancer. About 80% of all breast cancers are invasive ductal carcinomas. Invasive means that the cancer has 'invaded' or spread to the surrounding tissues. It also demonstrates the spread to liver.

Question 63:
Answer: b
Explanation: 80% reason for symptom of inappropriate anti-diuretic hormone syndrome (SIADH) is due to small cell lung cancer. Symptoms also include lethargy, muscle cramps and weakness.

Question 64:
Answer: d
Explanation: The symptoms such as acute pleuritic pain on left side, dyspnea, tachypnea, tachycardia, slight cough are consistent with Pneumothorax on left side. This occurs as a result of erosion of tumor through the surface of the lung. A tension Pneumothorax occurs with tracheal deviation when the air tries to escape. This requires immediate needle decompression and insertion of a chest tube.

Question 65:
Answer: a

Explanation: Symptoms for peripheral 3 neuropathy includes gradual onset of numbness, prickling or tingling in your feet or hands, which can spread upward into your legs and arms. Sharp, jabbing, throbbing or burning pain. Extreme sensitivity to touch. Therefore it is mandatory to teach proper home environments.

Question 66:
Answer: a
Explanation: When planning and developing educational material, it is important to consider the patient's physical, psychosocial and emotional needs.

Question 67:
Answer: a
Explanation: Multidisciplinary oncology care has been identified as a key enabler in the provision of high-quality treatment and care for cancer patients. Multidisciplinary teams aim at improving communication, coordination and decision making between the care professionals.

Question 68:
Answer: d
Explanation: The best action done by the nurse is to request the parents to leave a message for his son as it is a right of the patient to deny them from meeting him. The nurse cannot directly say the reason to the parents as it causes more worries to his parents. The nurse cannot either request the patient as it is his choice or talk with the hospice regarding this.

Question 69:
Answer: b

Explanation: Any applicant has to outline only about the job qualifications and requirements. The medical history should not be discussed till the job is offered. All the information regarding the insurance for future treatments and other enquiries has to be made only when their offer is confirmed. Only on any requirement, they can provide information about their cancer history and details.

Question 70:
Answer: b
Explanation: Before treating anxiety, it is important to know the causes of anxiety. The nurse must help in identifying the cause of anxiety as it has several risk factors.

Question 71:
Answer: a
Explanation: Skin breakdown occurs when blood flow to your skin is limited or cut off altogether. Left untreated, skin breakdown can lead to infection, amputation or even death.

Question 72:
Answer: a
Explanation: Pain associated with herpes zoster is described as continuous, deep and burning which can be severe and deliberating. Treatment for acute herpes zoster is by using opioids. Treatment for post herpetic neuralgia is tricyclic antidepressants.

Question 73
Answer: a
Explanation: Skin peeling can have causes that aren't due to underlying disease. Examples include sunburn, grass burn, prolonged time in water or prolonged skin contact with noxious liquid. Moisturizing skin cream can reduce dry desquamation.

Question 74:
Answer: b

Explanation: Carcinoid syndrome occurs when a rare cancerous tumor called a carcinoid tumor secretes certain chemicals into your bloodstream, causing a variety of signs and symptoms. Generally patients with age above 65 who have close relative relatives diagnosed with prostate cancer are said to have a higher risk for the development of neuroendocrine tumor and carcinoid syndrome.

Question 75:
Answer: c
Explanation: As leukopenia and thrombocytopenia are dose limiting toxicities that are not cumulative, therefore treatment cycle is between 22 to 28 days and recovers within 14 days.

Question 76

Answer: c
Explanation: Haloperidol is used to manage delirium. It is also used in the treatment of schizophrenia, tics in Tourette syndrome, mania in bipolar disorder, nausea and vomiting, delirium, agitation, acute psychosis.

Question 77:
Answer: d
Explanation: For about 15% patients receiving high dose of external beam radiation can cause radiation pneumonitis. With increased dyspnea and non productive cough, this can be characterized. Other symptoms include occurrence of blood while coughing(hemoptysis) in several places. The symptoms are evident on radiographs through ground glass opacification. This symptoms generally occur during the second or third month of the therapy. At certain cases, respiratory failure occurs.

Question 78:
Answer: a

Explanation: The vomit reflex of the patient can be avoided by having a deep breath and with controlled swallowing. The fluids should not be taken in large volume. Instead should be sipped in small amounts throughout the day.

Question 79:
Answer: a
Explanation: Stimulation is based generally on host cytotoxic and immunological response. Therefore the most common side effect will be the flu like symptoms.

Question 80:
Answer: d
Explanation: Bowel obstruction incident has been reported between 5.5% and 42% of patients with ovarian cancer. Symptoms include vomiting, distention, colicky pain, and diarrhea. However, signs of bowel movements depend on the location of obstruction. Medical treatment includes relieving the distention, correcting the fluid imbalances, and removing the source of the obstruction.

Question 81:
Answer: a
Explanation: An allogeneic stem cell transplant uses healthy blood stem cells from a donor to replace the disease or damaged region. This can vary between myeloablative and non myeloablative. This can cure acute lymphoblastic leukemia.

Question 82:
Answer: b
Explanation: The nurse should immediately discontinue the chemotherapeutic agent and monitor the patients respiratory and cardiovascular status as these symptoms are persistent with anaphylaxis. Dyspnea is generally treated with higher oxygen concentration and once the patient gets stabilized the corticosteroids and antihistamines can be administered in order to prevent the recurrence and to treat Urticaria and swelling.

Question 83:
Answer: a
Explanation: Monitoring the patient regarding the medication side effects can ensure proper treatment in advance. This can also be a precaution of any other side effects that can be caused due to other medicine with similar composition.

Question 84:
Answer: a
Explanation: Healthy communication can be established when the nurse is able to obtain information from the patient regarding the treatment process, understanding of the concepts and reaction to the treatment. This can promote more open and honest conversation between the patient and the nurse.

Question 85:
Answer: d
Explanation: Consumption of alcohol can lead to burning sensation of the mouth. It may also delay the healing process.

Question 86:
Answer: b
Explanation: There are several factors that affect weight of individual during chemotherapy. Therefore it is advisable to learn about the cause of weight loss from the patient through the heath care team.

Question 87:
Answer: c

Explanation: These are very common in cancer patients and occurs due to oral candidiasis. To treat and relieve this condition, nystatin oral suspension is used. If there is no cure of candidiasis then diflucan can be prescribed. During the night and after the meals dentures should be removed for cleansing. Tongue appears reddened causing irritation with disappearance of white lesions in some cases.

Question 88:
Answer: d
Explanation: Acetyl salicylic acid also known as aspirin generally reduces people's risk on cancer by frequent use. It is also said to reduce the mortality rate of gastrointestinal cancer.

Question 89:

Answer: d
Explanation: The cause of urine retention is due to the obstruction in the upper urinary tract. This appears secondary to the ovarian cancer. Michele is likely to developed uremia if she is unable to drain her urine as her ureters are obstructed. This is associated with hyperkalemia. The bladder tends to fill normally and gets distended with pain with any bladder injection or opioids induced deficiency of detrusor muscle contraction.

Question 90:
Answer: d
Explanation: Non harming or inflicting least harm is generally known as Nonmaleficence. This is to ensure least harm in order to bring more benefits. The actual act must be good or morally neutral with more positive benefits though it has negative effects also.

Question 91:
Answer: d

Explanation: Age appears to be a major factor in determining the risk of a patient regarding breast cancer. A mother who has been diagnosed with breast cancer at the age of 60 years of age is said to be facing a risk 2 to 4 times higher than that of those without these risk factors.

Question 92:
Answer: d
Explanation: Patients above the age of 60 years are at higher risk of graft-versus-host disease. This is because they had undergone an allogeneic transplant from a matched and unrelated donor.

Question 93:
Answer: b
Explanation: Michelle will be in a state where she is most likely to relate characters along with the test results. Survivor guilt occurs when a person tests negative and feel guilty as to why they were fortunate enough to test negative when a dear one tested positive.

Question 94:
Answer: b
Explanation: Staging is generally done in order to select the appropriate treatment for the cancer depending upon individual patient. It is categorized as pathological, biochemical, clinical and surgical and it's not a direct prediction method.

Question 95:
Answer: c
Explanation: The ASCO/ OND ensures the safety standards for the administration of chemotherapy. This generally conveys the staffing issue, chemotherapy planning preparation and administration.

Question 96:
Answer: b

Explanation: Using transvaginal ultrasound, BRCA1 or BRCA2 mutation patient must be screened every 6 months for ovarian cancer at the age of 25 along with Serum CA125 Level Checking. Michelle is advised for removal of ovaries and fallopian tube once she completes her child bearing or after 35 years of age.

Question 97:
Answer: b
Explanation: In order to plan efficiently for pain management, the oncology nurse and other members of the palliative care are advised to work along with the patient and their family.

Question 98
Answer: b
Explanation: Music therapy can be used for facilitating movement and overall physical rehabilitation and motivating clients to cope with treatment. It tends to reduce the duration of nausea and vomiting.

Question 99:
Answer: b
Explanation: Here oral contraceptive are recommended to aid in preventing the families from ovarian cancer, who have Lynch syndrome. Genetically they have no risk for breast cancer.

Question 100:
Answer: a
Explanation: Metastatic testicular tumors (nonseminomatous), Gestational trophoblastic neoplasm, locally recurrent or loco regional solid tumors (sarcomas, carcinomas and adenocarcinomas) Soft tissue sarcoma are some of the cancer for which Dactinomycin will be administered. It is considered a vesicant.

Question 101:
Answer: a

Explanation: Hand-foot syndrome is also called palmar-plantar erythrodysesthesia. It is a side effect of some cancer treatments. Hand-foot syndrome causes redness, swelling, and pain on the palms of the hands or on the soles of the feet. Sometimes blisters also appear.

Question 102:
Answer: b
Explanation: There is no harm in receiving the information from Rihanna regarding her sexual history in a non-judgmental and non-threatening manner. This shall help in receiving additional information in order to make a plan.

Question 103:
Answer: c
Explanation: Leukoreduction is the removal of white blood cells (or leukocytes) from the blood or blood components supplied for blood transfusion. After the removal of the leukocytes, the blood product is said to be Leukoreduced. Leukoreduced platelets are indicated for patients expecting multiple platelet transfusions to reduce the incidence of alloimmunization.

Question 104:
Answer: c
Explanation: Emphasizing functioning Vs dysfunction and capability Vs disabilities are certain rehabilitation principle. Balancing activity and rest time also emphasize the capability.

Question 105
Answer: c
Explanation: Improvement in successful adjustments include discussing her thoughts and feelings safely with an attentive and professional listener. So it is better to make the patient feel stress-free during the entire process.

Question 106:

Answer: b
Explanation: Anti-cancer medications and medications used to reduce side effects may contribute to the development of some eye problems such as photosensitivity.

Question 107
Answer: b
Explanation: Core concept of CQI: problems relate to process and variations in process lead to variation in result. Quality and success includes meeting or exceeding internal and external customer's need and expectations. This mainly focusses on 4 step loop process PLAN, DO, CHECK, ACT.

Question 108
Answer: c
Explanation: Darbepoetin Alfa injection is used to treat anemia (a lower than normal number of red blood cells). It generally causes progression in causing diseases with a decreased survival rate.

Question 109:
Answer: b
Explanation: The best way is to honor the patient's wish regarding the end of life care. In some cases, family members decide the patient's wish regardless of the patient's individual wish. And in other cases patients are unable to make any decisions. During these cases the health care providers and care givers are more aware of the patient's wish and therefore ensure that the patient's wish is honored.

Question 110:
Answer: b
Explanation: The important duty and responsibility is to inform the consent. The decision made should not depend on others and the patient should have the freedom of choice.

Question 111:

Answer: a
Explanation: Palmar plantar erythro dysesthesia is due to rupture of capillaries that generally occur while walking, or due to any activities that involves bearing extra weight.

Question 112:
Answer: c
Explanation: Change in the body structure can affect the psychologically. So it is better to let the patient express her feelings so that nurse can acknowledge the patient's loss and encourage her expression.

Question 113
Answer: a
Explanation: In order to deliver high amount of chemotherapy, intraperitoneal catheters or implanted ports are preferred highly for the patients with metastatic cancer into the abdomen and peritoneum, diagnosing ovarian cancer or colon mesothelioma or malignant ascites.

Question 114:
Answer: d
Explanation: Radiation therapy are received by non-surgical candidates due to impaired lung Function. This is generally curative for the patients with stage 1 and 2 cancer.

Question 115:
Answer: c
Explanation: Family members will grieve for the loss of their loved ones which is normal and expected reaction. Nurses can provide support to the family by validating the normal grief. Normal manifestations of grief include: sadness, anger, guilt, anxiety, loneliness, fatigue, helplessness, yearning, emancipation, relief, and numbness.

Question 116:

Answer: a
Explanation: By asking the patient about his or her importance can make the patient to focus on the goals while reframing hope. While some patients want to spend time with their family or complete any incomplete task while other patient will find this as a pain free. The nurse must help the patient along with the healthcare member to identify the patient's goal and should make sure that plans are made to make the patient achieve his or her goal.

Question 117
Answer: b
Explanation: By Administering Fluorouracil alone or in combination with other chemotherapy agent can increase the risk of mucositis.

Question 118:
Answer: a
Explanation: Skeletal-related events (SREs) are a common complication of bone metastases, and have serious negative consequences for patients with castrate-resistant prostate cancer (CRPC). Bone mineral loss and decreased testosterone from hormonal agents cause adverse skeletal events.

Question 119:
Answer: d
Explanation: After chemotherapy, certain side effects are being experienced by the patients. One such side effect is delayed Nausea, which occurs within 24 hours of chemotherapy and lasts up to 5 days.

Question 120:
Answer: a
Explanation: A breach of the duty of care occurs when one fails to fulfill his or her duty of care to act reasonably in some aspect.

Question 121:
Answer: b

Explanation: Survivor fears to change job because of loss of insurance. Survivors and their family are protected by ADA act (Americans with Disabilities Act).If insurance coverage is offered to all employees, it must be offered to the cancer survivor or the employer is in violation of the ADA as cancer is considered as disability according to ADA act.

Question 122:
Answer: c
Explanation: Cultural competence generally refers to the identification of differences in the culture, beliefs and respect those differences among different people throughout their treatment duration.

Question 123:
Answer: b
Explanation: Exposure of head and neck to radiation results in Hypothyroidism. This occurs when the thyroid produces insufficient amount of thyroid hormone. Risk increases with increased radiation dosage and for females. Symptoms generally include chronic fatigue, menstrual disturbances, hoarseness in voice, low pulse rate rate, thinning of hair and thickening of skin. It also causes some dementia with hypothyroidism.

Question 124:
Answer: a
Explanation: Irinotecan under the name of camptosar is a medication used to treat colon cancer, and small cell lung cancer. For colon cancer it is used either alone or with fluorouracil. For small cell lung cancer it is used with cisplatin. It is given by slow injection into a vein. About 35% of the people receiving this experience severe Diarrhea and neutropenia.

Question 125:
Answer: c

Explanation: These are said to be the consistent symptoms of SVCS due to invasion or compression of SVC, that are also associated with other cancer types such as breast, brain, resulting in cerebral anoxia, obstruction in bronchi and Laryngeal Edemas (at extreme cases) which can be treated by radiation, chemotherapy and surgery. Oxygen Therapy and corticosteroids are considered as supportive measures at extreme cases.

Question 126:
Answer: d
Explanation: Specialization and division of normal cells are promoted by proto oncogene. The change in genetic sequence can result in uncontrolled cell growth, that results in the formation of tumor. Transfer of proto oncogene to oncogene usually occurs in 3 ways: Point mutation, Translocation and Amplification.

Question 127:
Answer: c
Explanation: Descending colostomy location is in the left lower quadrant. Transverse colostomy has its position just below the waist line. Ascending colostomy location is in the right lower quadrant. Sigmoid colostomy is located in left upper quadrant.

Question 128:

Answer: d
Explanation: The nurse should be more responsible about the patient's feeling after hearing about the failure of treatment rather than reviewing the treatment possibility as prescribed by the physician.

Question 129
Answer: a

Explanation: The pain caused during the infusion of tamoxifen is due to tumor flare. The pain lasts only for a short duration and usually disappears with continuous therapy.

Question 130
Answer: a
Explanation: Anxiety disorders include panic attacks, obsessive-compulsive disorder and post-traumatic stress disorder. This can be reduced by mindfulness based stress reduction therapy.

Question 131
Answer: d
Explanation: Watson can probably balance his treatment with work schedules only if he is able to discuss his working hours with his officials and co-workers. Only with reduced work schedules and support from his work environment can facilitate smooth transition to workforce after treatment.

Question 132:
Answer: a
Explanation: Generally the family members of a dying patient find it difficult to identify the beneficial care that the patient requires. Therefore it is necessary for the nurse to coordinate the family members and provide support by clarifying doubts, educating family members and providing proper communication with the presence of health care officials.

Question 133:
Answer: a
Explanation: T2 N2 M1 is said to be the advanced metastatic cancer. It is said to be the stage 4 colon cancer. With an unresectable disease, cure is not possible. Until there is progression in disease, chemotherapy setting is given.

Question 134:
Answers: a

Explanation: The medications must be stopped as soon as the symptoms occur because vesicants such as anthracyclines cause local tissue damage and necrosis. The nurse must apply some ice to the area of administration to minimize the spread of the agent to the surrounding areas. The cold pack should be applied for 20 minutes for a minimum of four times daily for three days.

Question 135:
Answer: c
Explanation: Systemic inflammatory response syndrome (SIRS) is a generalized inflammatory response affecting many organ systems. A diagnosis of SIRS is made when two of the following is present: 1. Elevated (>38*
c) or subnormal rectal temperature (<36*c). 2. Tachypnea or paCo2<32 mm Hg 3. Tachycardia 4. Leukocytosis (>12,000)orleukopenia(<4000)

Question 136
Answer: d
Explanation: Carmustine also known as bis-chloroethylnitrosourea, BCNU, BiCNU is a medication used mainly for chemotherapy. It is a nitrogen mustard ÃŽ²-chloro-nitrosourea compound used as an alkylating agent. It generally causes pulmonary fibrosis.

Question 137:
Answer: a
Explanation: Success rates of hormonal therapy has been observed by treating breast cancer and prostate cancer.

Question 138:
Answer: d
Explanation: Lenalidomide is only available under the REVAssist® program to ensure patients are properly informed of fetal risks.

Question 139:
Answer: a

Explanation: The nurses should support only spiritual and cultural practices that are non-harming to patient's health

Question 140
Answer: d
Explanation: Prealbumin or transthyretin is monitored to determine changes in nutritional status. Prealbumin is said to be measured as it shows drastic decrease in level when there is a change in nutritional level. Albumin are said to be sensitive for long term protein deficiency rather than short term deficiency.

Question 141:
Answer: d
Explanation: According to the American Cancer Society Guidelines, in order to avoid average risk of prostate cancer in men, prostate specific antigen blood test has to be taken at the age of 50.

Question 142:
Answer: b
Explanation: Tacrolimus also known as protopoc and profag, is an immunosuppressive drug that is generally administered to a Robert after allogeneic organ transplant. This generally helps in lowering the risk of organ rejection.

Question 143:
Answer: b
Explanation: Lung cancer or Buccal cancer are said to cause higher risk of secondary malignancy affecting the skin and mucosa after completing the treatment for neck and head cancer.

Question 144:
Answer: c
Explanation: Despite progress in treating chemotherapy-induced nausea and vomiting (CINV), especially in the acute phase up to 24 hours after treatment, the condition is still one of the side effects in patient and delays in getting cured.

Question 145
Answer: b
Explanation: The mouse and human antibodies combine at a ratio of 70% human and 30% foreign antibodies. These are termed as chimeric monoclonal antibody.

Question 146
Answer: b
Explanation: The most predictive maladaptive response to the illness will be negative religious actions such as pleading the God for forgiveness, Passively deferring decision to God).

Question 147:
Answer: a
Explanation: Studies and researches confirm that there is a connection between the radon exposure and Lung Cancer. But there is no such studies confirming the link between breast bowel and bladder cancer with radon exposure.

Question 148:
Answer: c
Explanation: Lymphatic cancer is a risk to spinal cord compression that includes weakness in leg, loss of sensation and loss of urine or bowel control.

Question 149:
Answer: a
Explanation: Cell mediated immunity doesn't involve antibodies and they are mediated by the T cells and their cytokine products.

Question 150:
Answer: d

Explanation: Torsades de pointes is a specific form of polymorphic ventricular tachycardia in patients with a long QT interval. This also include few other life threatening reactions such as hepatocellular damage and allergic reactions

Question 151:
Answer: b
Explanation: In order to minimize the bleeding the patients are advised to wear shoes during ambulation in order to maintain skin integrity and avoid injury.

Question 152:

Answer: a
Explanation: Nurse has to ensure the privacy, safety, rights and confidentiality of patient details with respect and care by considering the environment of patients, articulate values and maintenance of professional integrity.

Question 153:
Answer: c
Explanation: Cancer cells are cells that divide relentlessly, forming solid tumors or flooding the blood with abnormal cells. Cell division is a normal process used by the body for growth and repair. They are characterized by uncontrolled movement and abnormal growth.

Question 154:
Answer: b
Explanations: Hydrating in order to prevent the renal injury is considered as one of the pretreatment guidelines of methotrexate.

Question 155
Answer: c

Explanation: The FDA is responsible for the protection of human subjects and it demands that when performing studies involving people, the researcher must obtain informed consent in easily understandable language. The informed consent must include all the necessary details as stated by the FDA.

Question 156:
Answer: b
Explanation: By tracking the expected bowel movements, patient can plan sexual activities easily depending on the bowel habits.

Question 157
Answer: c
Explanation: Successful treatment generally building up good rapport, ensuring cultural sensitivity with non-judgmental social and professional environmental. Therefore open communication about the therapy can provide informal support by the nurse to the patient and family members.

Question 158:
Answer: a
Explanation: Radiation can damage tissues by changing cell structure and damaging DNA. This can also lead to dimness in photophobia leading to Cataract.

Question 159:
Answer: a
Explanation: Metabolic abnormalities that are generally associated with tumor lysis syndrome which is an acute lymphocytic leukemia are Hyperkalemia, Hyperphosphatemia and Hypocalcemia.

Question 160:
Answer: b
Explanation: Repositioning in order to clear secretion can reduce the noise and rattled breathing caused by the dying patient.

Thank you for purchasing this book!

We know you could have picked any number of books to read, but you picked this book and for that we are extremely grateful.

What Do You Think of this OCN Exam Practise Questions Book?

We hope that this book added value and quality to your life and helped you in your OCN Exam preparation. If you liked this book and found some benefit in reading this, we'd like to hear from you and hope that you could take some time to post a review on Amazon. Your feedback and support will help us to greatly improve our writing for future projects and make this book even better.

Your review is very important to us as it helps us morally. Hope this book helped you in some way to crack the exam.

Warm Regards,
OCN Exam Expert Team

www.ingramcontent.com/pod-product-compliance
Lightning Source LLC
Chambersburg PA
CBHW052336220526
45472CB00001B/449